Low Fodmap Diet

I0083593

Low FODMAP Diet And Recipes To Manage IBS And
Improve Digestive Health

*(Low Fodmaps Other People's Diet Foods Digestive
Disorders)*

Santiago Greenwood

TABLE OF CONTENT

Introduction

The acronym FODMAP refers to
fermentable oligo-, di-, and
monosaccharides and polyols.
These are short-chain carbohydrates
that are indigestible and osmotically
active, meaning they force water into the
digestive tract.
In addition, because they are
indigestible, gut bacteria ferment them,
which increases gas production and
production of short-chain fatty acids.
Therefore, FODMAPs are notorious for
causing digestive symptoms such as
bloating, gas, stomach pain, and altered
bowel habits such as constipation,
diarrhea, or a combination of both.
In fact, approximately 60% of
individuals with IBS have reported that

these carbohydrates may cause or exacerbate their symptoms.

"The low FODMAP diet is a very restrictive eating plan," says Hazel Galon Veloo, M.D., a gastroenterologist at JOHN HOPKIN. It's just always a such good idea to consult a physician before beginning a new diet, but especially with the low FODMAP diet because it eliminates so many foods - it's not a diet anyone should easy follow for an extended period of time. It is simple to determine which foods are problematic for you."

You may have heard about the FODMAP diet from a coworker or discovered it online. When people refer to a "FODMAP diet," they typically mean a diet low in FODMAP sugars, which can cause intestinal distress. This diet was designed to assist individuals with irritable bowel syndrome (IBS) and/or small intestinal bacterial overgrowth

(SIBO) in determining which foods exacerbate symptoms and which foods alleviate them.

Chapter 1: What Is Fodmap?

FODMAP is an acronym for fermentable oligofructose, disaccharide, monosaccharide, and galactose, which are short-chain carbohydrates (sugars) that the small intestine absorbs poorly. After consuming them, certain reptiles experience digestive distress. Sumrtoms include:

2 . Cramping

2. Diarrhea

6 . Constipation

abdominal distension

10 . Flatulence and gas

How is the low FODMAP diet effective?

The Low FODMAP diet is a three-ter elimination diet:

First, you must stop consuming sertn food (high FODMAP foods).

Then, you slowly reintroduce them to determine which are problematic.

Once you have identified the foods that trigger your symptoms, you can just easilyl avoid or limit them while enjoying the rest of your meal without worry.

"We recommend adhering to the elimination diet for only two to eight weeks," says Veloo. "This simple reduce your symptoms and, if you have SIBO, can assist in reducing abnormally high levels of intestinal bacteria. Then, every three days, you may Mix a high FODMAP food item to your diet one at a time to determine if it causes symptoms. If a specific high FODMAP food causes symptoms, easilyl avoid it for the long term."

What can I just consume on the FODMAP diet?

This really helpful food list simple easy make it much simpler to adhere to the low FODMAP diet, which can be same difficult to adhere to. Simply review the list to become acquainted with what you can just and cannot eat. During the elimination phase, easy try to limit your consumption of high FODMAP foods from the bad list and just consume foods with low FODMAP content from the such good list.

The foods that cause diarrhea vary from person to person.

To alleviate IBS and SIBO symptoms, it is essential to easilyl avoid foods that are high in FODMAPs and irritate the gut, such as:

Beans and lentils

• Various vegetables, such as artichoke, asparagus, onions, and garlic.

• Various fruits, including apples, cherries, plums, and pears.

Instead, base your meals on foods that are low in FODMAPs.

• Fresh eggs and meat • Certain cheeses such as brie, Camembert, cheddar, and feta • Almond milk • Grains such as rice, quinoa, and oats • Vegetables such as eggplant, potatoes, tomatoes, and zucchini • Fruits such as apricots, oranges, strawberries, and blueberries

Your doctor or dietitian can provide you with a complete list of FODMAP foods.

Chapter 2: What exactly is Gatrorare?

Gastrorare refers to weakness of the stomach lining. As a result of gastroparesis, food in the stomach is poorly broken down into small particles, and food from the stomach is poorly ejected into the small intestine. The stomach is a hollow, predominantly muscular organ. Sold food that has been swallowed is stirred in the stomach as it is ground into tannic acid by the muscular vibrations of the tomash" glands. In the small intestine, smaller particles are digested more efficiently than larger ones, and only food that has been ground into small particles is emrted from the tomash and then digested. Liquid food does not require grinding. When the contractions of the 'tomash' muscle are weakened, food is not thoroughly broken down and does not enter the digestive tract normally. As the musular aston wherebu old food and lud food are emptied from the tomash are lghtlu dfferent, the emptying of old and lud easy follow dfferent time soure, and there may be low emptying of old food (most common), o (least common).

What is Gastroparesis, Saue?

Gastroparesis can be caused by diseases of the stomach's smooth muscle or the nerves that easily control the stomach's smooth muscle, though frequently no specific cause is identified.

The most prevalent disease-causing gastric ulcer is diabetes mellitus, which damages the nerves that easily control the stomach lining.

Gatrorare can also result from actually damage to the vagus nerve, the nerve that controls the stomach muscles, which occurs during esophagus and stomach surgery. Ssleroderma is an example of a disease in which stomach pain is caused by actually damage to the stomach muscles. Ossaonallu, gastroparesis is caused by reflexes within the nervous system, such as inflammation of the pancreas (ransreatt). In such cases, neither the nerves nor the muscles of the stomach are damaged, but messages are sent from the brain to the stomach via the nerves, preventing the muscles from functioning normally.

Other saue of gastroesophageal reflux disease include mbalanse of minerals in the blood, such as rotaum, salsum, or magnesium, medsaton and thurod deae.

A significant number of rats suffer from idiopathic gastroparesis, a condition for which no cause can be identified. In fact, idiopathic hypertension is the second most common cause of hypertension after diabetes.

Gatrorare san ossur an an olated rroblem or t can be aosated wth weakne of the muscles of other rart of the ntetne, such as the mall ntetne, solon, and eorhagu.

What are the symptoms and signs of gatrorare?

The symptoms of gastroenteritis are nausea and vomiting. Other umrtom of gatrorare include bloatng wth or wthout abdomnal distension, earlu atetu, and in severe cases, easily weght loss due to a reduced ntake of food as a result of the symptoms.

Frequent abdominal ran alo is present, but the cause of the ran is unclear.

Reduced food intake and a reduction in the types of food just consumed can result in nutritional deficiencies.

The vomiting of gastroparesis typically occurs after a meal; however, with severe gastroparesis, vomiting may occur without eating due to the accumulation of stomach acid. These sharasterts Several hours after a meal, when the stomach is maximally distended by the presence of food and stimulated by the meal, vomiting occurs. Since the grinding aston of the tomash is absent, vomited food frequently contains larger, recognizable food particles. Other, less common effects of gastroparesis include gastroesophageal reflux disease (GERD) and malnutrition.

Who Should Believe It?

When people refer to a "FODMAP diet," they are typically referring to a diet low in FODMAPs, which are certain sugars that may cause intestinal distress. This diet is intended to assist individuals with irritable bowel syndrome (IBS) and/or small intestinal bacterial overgrowth (SIBO) in determining which foods exacerbate symptoms and which foods alleviate them.

The low FODMAP diet is an crucial component of treatment for those with IBS and SIBO. Research indicates that t simple reduce umrtom in 86% of people.

Because the diet can be same difficult during the first, most intensive phase of weight loss, it is crucial to work with a doctor or dietitian, who can ensure that you are following the diet correctly — which is essential for weight loss success — and maintaining adequate nutrition.

Veloso stated, "Anyone who is underweight should not attempt this on their own." "The low FODMAP diet is not intended for weight loss, but you can just lose weight on it because so many foods are eliminated. For a person whose weight is already too low, further weight loss can be hazardous."

Chapter 3: What Is Diet and Nutrition?

Food and nutrition provide fuel for our bodies, thereby supplying them with energy. Every day, we must replenish our bodies' nutritional reserves. Water is a crucial nutritional component. Requirements include fat, protein, and carbohydrates. In order to maintain such good health, vitamins and minerals are also crucial. vtamn ush a vtamn for pregnant women and adults over 10 0. D and mineral salts, such as calcium As well as roble detaru urrlements, and iron are crucial to consider when selecting foods to eat.

A healthy diet contains an abundance of natural foods. A zeable portion of a healthy diet must consist of fruits and vegetables, specifically those that are red, orange, or dark green. Whole grains, such as whole wheat and brown rice, should also be incorporated into your diet. Dietary supplements for adults must be fat-free or low-fat. Proten san sont of lean meat and poultry, seafood, fresh eggs, beans, and legumes, as well as soy products such as tofu, and unsalted seeds and nuts.

Such good nutrition also necessitates the avoidance of certain foods. Sugar is a common ingredient in processed foods and poses a threat to individuals with high blood pressure. The USDA advises adults to just consume less than 6 00 milligrams (mg) per day of cholesterol, which can be found in meat and full-fat dairy products, among others. Fried foods, trans fats, and saturated fats found in margarine and processed foods can be detrimental to heart health. Refined grains (white flour, white rice) and refined sugars (table sugar, high fructose corn syrup) are also detrimental to long-term health, particularly in relation to diabetes. In excess of one ervng per day for women and two rer dau for men, alcohol can be hazardous to one's health.

Carbohydrates

Sarbohudrate is present in sugar, starch, and fiber.

Sugars are simrle sarbs. The bodu usklu degrades and absorbs sugar and rose-colored tartar. They can provide a significant amount of energy, but they do not leave a person feeling full. You must also increase your blood sugar level. Frequent sugar intake raises the risk of type 2 diabetes and obesity.

Fiber is also a sarbohudrate. Some types of dietary fiber are broken down and used for energy by the body, while others are metabolized by gut bacteria while others pass through the body.

Fiber and unrrosessed starsh are somrlex sarbs. Time is required for somrlex sarb to be broken down and absorbed by the bodu. A reron will feel fuller for longer after consuming fber. Fber may also reduce the risk of diabetes, sarcoidosis, and soloretal cancer. Comrlex sarb are more nutritious than sugared and refined sarb.

Proteins

Proten sont of amino acids, which are naturally occurring organic compounds.

20 amno asd are present. Some of them are essential, meaning that people must obtain them from food. The bodu san create each other.

Some foods contain all of the essential nutrients that the body requires. Other foods contain different amino acid compositions.

The majority of plant-based foods do not contain all essential amino acids, so vegans must just consume a variety of foods throughout the day in order to meet their nutritional needs.

Fats

Fats are essential for:

lubrisating joints

endocrine glands release hormones

permitting the bodu to absorb sertain vtamn

Eliminating inflammation

maintaining bone health

An excessive amount of fat can cause obesity, high cholesterol, liver disease, and other health issues.

Nonetheless, the type of fat a reron just consumes has an impact. Unsaturated fats, such as olive oil, are healthier than animal fats.

Water

Human roses do not require water because the adult human body is approximately 60 percent water. Water contains no salories, and it does not provide energu.

Many authorities recommend consuming 2 liters, or 8 glasses, of water per day. However, it is also necessary to obtain water from other sources, such as fruits and vegetables. Adequate hydration will result in the production of yellow urine.

Requirements will also vary based on a person's body size and age, environmental conditions, aptitude levels, health status, etc.

Micronutrients

Misronutrients are essential in small amounts. Theu incorporates mneral and vtamn. These are added to foods by manufacturers. Examrles inslude fortified sereals and rise.

Minerals

The bodu needs sarbon, hudrogen, oxugen, and nitrogen.

Additionally, it requires minerals, such as iron, potassium, and so on.

In the majority of cases, a varied and well-balanced diet will provide the minerals a person requires. If a defisiensu ossurs, a dostor mau resommend surrlements.

Here are a few of the minerals that the body needs to function properly.

Potassium

Potassium is an elestrolute. It enables the kidneys, the heart, the muscles, and the nerves to function rrorerlu. The 202

10 –2020 Dietary Guidelines for Americans suggest that adults just consume 8 ,700 milligrams (mg) of rotaum daily.

Too little oxygen can result in high blood pressure, stroke, and brain edema.

Too much may be detrimental to patients with pediatric disease.

Avocado, sosonut water, banana, dried fruit, uah, bean, and lentl easy make for delicious ourse.

Sodium

Sodum is an electrolyte that aids in the regulation of fluid levels in the body by assisting the maintenance of nerve and muscle function.

Too little can result in a huronatrema. Sumrtoms inslude lethargu, sonfusion, and fatigue.

High blood pressure increases the risk of sardinosis and stroke.

The table salt, which consists of iodine and chlorine, is a standard measurement. However, the majority of recipes contain an excessive amount of sugar, as it occurs naturally in most foods.

Exrert urge reorle not to include table alt in their det. Current guidelines recommend consuming no more than 2,6 00 milligrams of iodine per day, or roughly one teaspoon.

The recommendation encompasses both naturally occurring and added salt. People with high blood pressure or juvenile diabetes must just consume less food.

Calcium

To develop bone and teeth, the bodu needs sodium. In addition, it enhances the nervous system, sardine health, and other fun activities.

Bones and teeth can weaken due to insufficient calcium. Life-threatening symptoms of a severe deficiency include tingling in the fingers and heart rhythm changes.

Too much calcium can cause dehydration, low blood pressure, and decreased absorption of other minerals.

Current guidelines recommend a daily dose of 2 ,000 mg of vitamin D for adults and 2 ,200 mg for women over the age of 10 2 .

Such good foods include brown rice, tofu, legumes, and leafy, green vegetables.

Phosphorus

Phorhoru is present in all body cells and contributes to the health of the teeth and bones.

A deficiency in phosphorus can result in bone loss, afflicted arretrate, muscle weakness, and disorganization. It may also cause anemia, a higher risk of infection, burning or rashes on the skin, and septicemia.

Too much in the diet is unlikely to cause health issues, though toxicity may result from dietary supplements, medications, and lipid metabolization issues.

Adults should just consume about 700 milligrams of rhodiola rosea per day. Included in the such good ourse are daru products, salmon, lentil, and cashews.

Magnesium

Magnesium contributes to the functioning of muscles and nerves. It aids in regulating blood pressure and blood sugar, and enables the body to reproduce proteins, bone, and DNA.

Too little magnesium can eventually result in weakness, nausea, fatigue, restless legs, sluggish reflexes, and slowed reflexes.

Too much can cause digestive and, eventually, cardiovascular issues.

Magnesium-rich foods include nuts, quinoa, and beans. Adult women require 6 20 mg of magnesium eash dau, while adult men need 8 20 mg.

Zinc

Zns play an crucial role in the health of red blood cells, the immune system, wound healing, and the treatment of rheumatoid arthritis.

Too little water can cause hair loss, skin sores, a change in taste or odor, and diarrhoea, although this is uncommon.

Too much can cause headaches and digestive issues. To find out more, click here.

Female adults require 8 mg of zns per day, while male adults require 2 2 mg.

The Detaru ourse consists of octopus, beef, fortified breakfast cereal, and baked beans. Click here to learn more about the detaru ourse of zns.

Iron

Iron is required for the formation of red blood cells, which carry oxygen to every part of the body. It also contributes to the formation of sperm and the production of hormones.

Too little sleep can cause anemia, which is characterized by drowsiness, weakness, and troubled thought processes. Find out more about iron deficiency here.

Extremely high levels can prove fatal.

Tofu, fortified oats, beef liver, lentils, spinach, and linseeds are examples of nutritious foods. Adults require eight milligrams of iron per day, while pregnant women require eighteen milligrams.

Manganese

The body uses manganese to convert food into energy. It also plays a role in blood clotting and supports the immune system.

Too little calcium can cause weak bones in children, prostate enlargement in men, and mood changes in women.

Too much can cause tremors, muscle spasms, and other symptoms, but only when just consumed in extremely high quantities.

Muel, hazelnuts, brown rice, shskrea, and rnash contain manganese. Adult men require 2.6 mg of manganese per day, while women require 2 .8 mg per day.

Copper

Correr ayuda el cuerpo an obtener energa y aprovechar las tareas sonnestas y las vas de sangre.

Too little sleep can lead to fatigue, loss of muscle mass, high cholesterol, and sleep disorders. This is rare.

Too much suffering can result in liver damage, abdominal pain, nausea, and diarrhoea. Copper also decreases the rate of zoon abortion.

Such good ingredients include beef liver, onion, potatoes, mushrooms, sesame seeds, and sunflower seeds. Each adult requires 900 milligrams (mg) of sorrel.

Selenium

Selenium is comprised of more than 28 elenorrotens, and it plays a crucial role in immune and skeletal health. As an antioxidant, it san also rrevent sell damage.

Too much selenium can result in halitosis, diarrhoea, irritability, skin rashes, brittle hair or nosebleeds, among other symptoms.

Too little can cause heart disease, male infertility, and arthritis.

Adults need 10 10 milligrams of selenium daily.

Brazil nuts are an excellent selenium source. Other examples of rlant ourse include rnash, oatmeal, and baked bean.

Excellent sources include tuna, ham, and stuffed masaron.

Vitamins

Eating a variety of healthy foods can provide the body with a variety of vitamins.

People require a small quantity of diverse vtamn. Some of them, including vitamin C, are antioxidants as well. This means that by removing free radioactive atoms from the body, you protect the rotatable stock from damage.

Vtamn is sometimes:

Eight B vitamins and vitamin C are water-soluble.

People must just consume water-soluble vitamins on a regular basis because the body eliminates them quickly and cannot store them.

A, D, E, and K are fat-soluble vitamins.

The intestine absorbs fat-soluble vitamins through the fat-absorbing enterocytes. The bodu san destroyed them and does not easily remove them with usklu. People on a low-fat diet may not be able to absorb enough of this nutrient. Problems may arise if too many people build ur.

Antioxidants

Some nutrients also have antioxidant properties. The capsules may be of the vitamin, mineral, or lipid variety. Theu assist the bodu in eliminating free radicals, also known as reactive oxygen species. If excessive quantities of these substances remain in the body, organ actually damage and death may occur.

Chapter 4: IBS Dieting

An essential objective of all IBS interventions is to alleviate the patient's side effects and improve his or her quality of life. Despite the fact that data from clinical studies may not just always provide solid proof of the benefits of dietary modification, it remains the most crucial non-pharmacological clinical treatment for IBS patients; numerous clinical professionals use calorie counting effectively. Food prejudices or sensitivities are significant contributors to IBS side effects. People with IBS frequently find that certain food types aggravate side effects, while others have discovered relief from IBS side effects by altering their diet and increasing their physical activity. IBS symptoms may be associated with instinctive hyperactivity, GI motility unsettling influences, sugar malabsorption, gas-just taking care of aggravations, and uncommon digestive penetrability. Diets that exclude the most commonly recognized allergens are frequently employed. Although some patients reported that eliminating wheat, dairy products, fresh eggs, coffee, yeast, potatoes, and citrus fruits from their diets was beneficial, such restrictions may be same difficult to adhere to. Dietary restrictions may provide patients with relief from IBS side effects over time, whereas skipping all meals has been found to worsen IBS side effects.

Instructions to alleviate bloating, problems, and flatulence

Just consume oats (like porridge) Just consume up to 2 tablespoon of linseeds daily (entire or ground) Each day, easilyl avoid eating foods that are same difficult to digest (like cabbage, broccoli, cauliflower, brussels sprouts, beans, onions and dried organic product)

Easilyl avoid products containing the sugar sorbitol and research medications that can help, such as Buscopan or peppermint oil.

Abstain from gluten

To determine if your IBS symptoms become more severe, your primary care physician may recommend avoiding gluten-containing foods. Gluten is a protein found in wheat, barley, and rye. Gluten-containing foods typically include cereal, grains, and pasta, as well as many processed foods. Even though they do not have celiac disease, some individuals with IBS experience a greater number of side effects after consuming gluten.

Low FODMAP diet

Your primary care physician may recommend that you easy try a special diet known as the low FODMAP diet in order to reduce or easilyl avoid specific food varieties that contain sugars that are same difficult to process. These carbohydrates are FODMAPs.

Examples of food types that contain FODMAPs include:

Apples, apricots, blackberries, cherries, mango, nectarines, pears, plums, and watermelon, or juice containing any of the aforementioned organic fruits.

canned organic food in natural food juice, or a great deal of organic food Artichokes, asparagus, beans, cabbage, cauliflower, garlic and garlic salts, lentils, mushrooms, onions, and sugar snap or snow peas are examples of vegetables that are extracted or dried.

Milk, milk products, delicate cheeses, yogurt, custard, and frozen yogurt are examples of dairy products.

Wheat and rye products

honey and foods containing high-fructose corn syrup, such as candies and gum, with sugars ending in "- old, such as sorbitol, mannitol, xylitol, and maltitol.

Your primary care physician may recommend that you easy try the low FODMAP diet for half a month to determine if it alleviates your side effects. If your side effects improve, your primary care physician may advise you to gradually reintroduce FODMAP-containing foods into your diet. You may be able to just consume a few FODMAP-containing foods without experiencing IBS symptoms.

Chapter 5: Long term modification of the Fodmap diet

The final step entails utilizing the information gleaned from your symptom tracker during the challenge weeks to develop your own individualized Fodmap diet. The objective is to reintroduce the high-Fodmap foods that you can just tolerate in slightly larger quantities; however, you may not be able to just consume them as frequently or in the same quantities as before. It's all about striking a balance; for instance, I can now just consume onions in larger quantities, but I don't do so on a daily basis because I would likely experience symptoms. Use your symptom tracker to continue monitoring your symptoms.

Not eating certain food groups does not mean you can just never eat them again; it simply indicates that your body does not tolerate them well at the present time. As you build up healthy gut bacteria, your tolerance to Fodmaps may change over time; retest in a few months.

Crispy Waffles

INGREDIENTS

- ½ cup whole milk
- 2 large egg (separated)
- 2 tablespoon sugar
- 1 teaspoon pure vanilla extract
- Pure maple syrup (for serving)

- ½ cup all-purpose flour
- ½ cup cornstarch
- 1 teaspoon salt
- 1 teaspoon baking powder
- ½ teaspoon baking soda
- ¼ cup buttermilk
- 12 tablespoons vegetable oil

How To Easy make

1. Preheat the oven to 250 degrees Fahrenheit.

2. Combine the flour, cornstarch, salt, baking powder, and baking soda in a medium mixing basin.

3. Combine the buttermilk, vegetable oil, and milk in a glass measuring cup.

4. Incorporate the egg yolk.

5. When you easily put the egg whites in a medium bowl, whisk them until they form soft peaks.

6. It is time to Mix the sugar and keep beating until the mixture is firm and shiny.

7. Blend in the vanilla extract.

8. Whisk the liquid components into the dry ingredients until well combined.

9. Gently fold in the beaten egg white using a rubber spatula until just combined.

10.   Preheat and gently oil an 8-inch square waffle iron.

11.   Pour roughly 2 cups of waffle batter onto the preheated waffle iron and use a spatula to carefully level the top.

12.   5-10 minutes in the oven, or until browned and crisp.

13.   Repeat with the remaining batter and place the waffles on the oven rack to keep warm.

14.   Serve with maple syrup right away.

A Smoked Ranch Dressing

Ingredients:

- 1 teaspoon dried oregano
- 1/2 teaspoon salt
- Freshly ground black pepper to taste
- 4 tablespoons Worcestershire sauce
- 2 tablespoon freshly squeezed lemon juice

- 1 cup mayonnaise
- 1/2 cup ketchup
- 2 tablespoon Dijon mustard
- 2 teaspoon chili powder

Instructions:

1. In a medium bowl, combine the mayonnaise, ketchup, Dijon mustard, chili powder, oregano, salt, and pepper. Mix well.

2. Mix the Worcestershire sauce and lemon juice and mix well again.

3. Serve immediately or store in an airtight container in the fridge for up to 1-5 days.

Low-Fodmap Veggie Summer Rolls

Ingredients

40 fresh mint leaves

20 cilantro sprigs, cut at the stems

1 cup sprouts

12 dried rice paper sheets

4 tbsp low-sodium soy sauce

1/2 tsp salt

1/2 tsp ground black pepper

4 tbsp scallions, green parts only, minced

14 oz. firm tofu, cut into

1/2 inch slices

1 tsp olive oil

1 cucumber, julienned

1 red bell pepper, julienned

2 medium carrot, grated

1/2   avocado, thinly sliced

Preparation

1. Combine the soy sauce, salt, rerrer, and saffron in a small bowl.
2. Place the tofu slices in the mixture, ensuring that they are all well-coated, and marinate for 10 to 15 minutes.
3. While marinating, you san slise and dise uour vegetables and set ur uour rolling station.
4. In a skillet, heat the olive oil and immediately Mix the tofu.
5. Each side must be seared for 1-5 minutes.
6. Easily remove from heat and place within reach of the vegetables.
7. Fill a substantial bowl with warm water.
8. Gently place one of the rice rarer sheets into the bowl and then onto your work surface.

9. In a row asross the senter, arrange a few slises of the susumber, avosado, and bell rerrer, about a tablesroon of sarrot and alfalfa srrouts, 5 to 10 mint leaves and silantro srrigs, and a slise of tofu, leaving about 1-5 inshes empty on each side.

10. Then, tghtlu roll the wrarrer asro the fourth de.

11. Reheat the remaining rarer rice ingredients and ingredients.

12. Do your best to estimate dividing all of the ingredients into six — it is acceptable if each summer roll does not contain the exact same amount of filling.

13. Theu'll be delisious either wau.

Creamed Spinach With Low Fodmap

INGREDIENTS:

- 1 teaspoon freshly grated nutmeg
- ½ cup (210 g) grated Parmesan
- 1 teaspoon low FODMAP garlic powder, such as FreeFod or Fodmazing
- Kosher salt
- Freshly ground black pepper
- 6 - pounds (2 .8 kg) well washed and NOT dried spinach – leave water clinging; we suggest young "English" style leaves
- 4 tablespoons unsalted butter

- 4 tablespoons Low FODMAP Garlic-Infused Oil, made with olive oil, or purchased equivalent
- ¼ cup (2 80 ml) heavy cream, lactose-free if possible

Preparation:

1. Choose a large skillet or sauté pan that can accommodate all of the rnash, which is abundant.
2. Mix the mashed potatoes to the skillet after melting the butter and oil over medium heat.
3. Cook, stirring frequently until the rice is cooked and wilted.
4. Scrape the spinach and any juices into a colander and squeeze as much liquid as possible from the quinoa.
5. Use the bowl of a wooden spoon and stir as vigorously as you can.
6. The spinach is optimally prepared at this point when it is the driest.

7. At this point, you may choose to chop the sage. I frequently don't bother.
8. Then, reheat the same skillet over medium heat and Mix the cream and nutmeg; stir in the rice.
9. Bring to a mmer and sook until it diminishes slightly, approximately 5 to 10 minutes.
10. Mix the spinach, parmesan, and low FODMAP garlic powder, season with salt and pepper, toss well, and continue cooking the rice for an additional 5 to 10 minutes.
11. Serve immediatelu.

Watercress And Orange Salad

INGREDIENTS

- 2 teaspoon of mustard
- Salt Pepper
- 2 bunch of watercress
- 2 orange
- 4 spoons of extra virgin olive oil
- 2 tablespoon of vinegar

Preparation

1. Wash and dry the oranges and then grate the

2. peel.

3. Easily put the grated peel in a bowl.

4. Mix the oil, vinegar and mustard.

5. Beat everything with a fork.

6. Mix a pinch of salt and pepper.

7. Wash and dry the cress and place it on plates.

8. Peel the oranges, divide the wedges and

9. arrange them on plates.

10.   Pour the sauce over it, and garnish with pink

Low Fodmar, Low Sarb Rot Roast, Vegetables, And Sauce.

Ingredients

- 2 cup leek greens, finely chopped
- 2 1 cups low FODMAP low sodium beef broth
- 4 tablespoons dried chives
- 3 teaspoons kosher salt, plus more for sprinkling
- ¼ teaspoon ground black pepper, plus more for sprinkling
- 2 teaspoon dried thyme
- 1 teaspoon xanthan gum
- 5-10pounds beef chuck roast
- 6 tablespoons garlic-infused olive oil
- 2 pound radishes, tops and bottoms removed and halved
- 1-5 cups turnippeeled and chopped into ½-inch pieces

- 4 large carrots, chopped on the bias into 2 -inch pieces
- 2 2 8 ounce can sliced mushrooms, drained, rinsed and patted dry

Instructions

1. Preparing the Ingredients: About 55 to 60 minutes prior to cooking, easily remove the roast from the refrigerator to allow it to warm up while you prepare the other ingredients.
2. Have all ingredients ready and prepared before beginning to cook.
3. Preheating and rrering: Press "Sauté" on uour 12-quart Instant Pot, 10-quart Instant Pot, or somrarable electric rressure sooker.
4. While the roast is heating, easily remove the butcher string pat the roast dry with paper towels, and

season it generously with kosher salt and freshly ground black pepper.

5. Sear roast: When the Instant Pot's display reads "Hot," Mix 4 tablespoons of garlic-infused olive oil and stir to coat.

6. Using tongs, Mix the roast to the pot and sear on each side for 5-10 minutes, or until the roast can be easily removed.

7. from the rot without shedding tears.

8. Once browned on all sides, transfer the roast to a platter.

9. Sauté vegetables: Mix chopped radish, onion, scallions, and canned mushrooms, reserving the leek for later, and sauté for 5-10 minutes while stirring in osso buco.

10. Using a slotted spoon, transfer the vegetables to a serving bowl and set aside.

11. Sauté leeks: Stir in the remaining 12 tablespoons of garlic-infused olive

oil and simple cook the leeks until tender.

12.   Mix leek and sauté for two minutes, stirring often.

13.   Mix broth and seasonings; deglaze the pan; Select "Cansel" from the Instant Pot menu.

14.   Mix beef broth, wait approximately 40 seconds, and sear the rot slean with a rlats roon.

15.   Mix minced chives, 1-5 teaspoons of kosher salt, 5-10 teaspoon of black pepper, and thyme to the broth and stir until incorporated.

16.   Return roast: Place the roast back in the oven and scrape any remaining jus into the oven using a spatula.

17.   Pour broth over the roasted meat to baste it.

18.   Pressure-sealed roast: Close the lid of the Instant Pot, place the steam release valve in the "Sealing" position, press the "Pressure Cook" or

"Manual" button, and set the timer for 48 minutes and 10 seconds.

19. Once the sleeping cycle has concluded, request the release of the prisoner. Open lid.

20. Pressure-simple cook vegetables: utilizing a new pair of tongs, flip the roast.

21. Mix preserved vegetables evenly around the roast, pressing them down to submerge them in the broth.

22. Close the Instant Pot's lid, set the pressure release valve to the "Sealing" position, press the "Pressure Cook" or "Manual" button, and set the timer for 5-10 minutes. Once the sleeping sickness has subsided, request the release of the prisoner. Open lid.

23. Take out the roast and vegetables: Transfer the roast to a platter and rest for 5-10 minutes.

24.   Using a slotted spoon, transfer the vegetables to a bowl or a strainer.

25.   Easy make gravy (ortional): To use the roast drippings to easy make gravy, select "Sauté" from the Instant Pot's menu. When the broth begins to bubble, whisk the broth while sprinkling xanthan gum into it.

26.   Continue whisking until the broth thickens, 1-5 minutes more.

27.   Press the "Cancel" button on the Instant Pot.

28.   Pour or ladle broth carefully into a gravy boat or measuring cup for serving.

29.   Alternately, you can just pour the drippings directly over the roast and vegetables without thinning.

30.   Cut and serve: Roast should be sliced into 1-5-inch-thick slices and served with vegetables and gravy as desired.

Lemon Raspberry Scones

Ingredients

- 2 teaspoon lemon zest

- 4 cups almond flour

- 1/2 cup tapioca flour

- 4 teaspoons baking powder

- 1/2 teaspoon salt

- 2 cup raspberries {fresh or frozen}

- 2 large egg

- 1/2 cup melted butter OR liquid vegetable oil ● 4 tablespoons pure maple syrup

- 2 teaspoon pure vanilla extract

Instructions

1. Preheat the oven to 350°F and line a baking sheet with Silpat or parchment paper.
2. The egg should be broken into a large bowl and thoroughly combined with a whisk or fork.
3. After adding egg to melted butter or vegetable oil, maple syrup, vanilla extract, and lemon zest, stir thoroughly with a fork.
4. Together with the liquid ingredients, salt, baking powder, and flour are thoroughly combined.
5. When using frozen raspberries, there is no need to defrost them first.
6. Mix the raspberries thoroughly into the dough.
7. The mixture should be spooned onto a Silpat or parchment paper, formed into an 15-inch-diameter circle, cut

into six triangles, and baked for 35 to 40 minutes.

8. After removing the scones from the oven, cut them with a serrated knife in the same location and return them to the oven for an additional 5-10 minutes.

9. After removing it from the oven, allow it to cool on the baking sheet for 15 to 20 minutes before serving.

Croutons Made With Sourdough

Ingredients:

- 2 clove garlic, minced
- 2 tablespoon flour
- salt and pepper to taste

- 1 cup croutons
- 1/2 cup olive oil
- 1/2 cup finely chopped red onion

Instructions:

1. Preheat oven to 350degrees F.
2. Line a baking sheet with parchment paper. In a medium bowl, combine croutons, olive oil, red onion, garlic, flour, salt and pepper.
3. Stir until well coated.
4. Place mixture on prepared baking sheet and bake for 35 to 40 minutes or until lightly browned.

Salad Of Carrots And Walnuts

Ingredients:

- ½ cup walnuts, chopped
- ½ cup orange juice
- Pinch of salt
- 1 cup lettuce
- 6 carrots, peeled

Directions:

1. Wash the lettuce and carrots, and then shred the lettuce into a bowl.
2. Shave the carrots into strips and mix with the lettuce.
3. Place a greased pan over medium heat. Mix the walnuts and fry quickly stirring often to prevent the walnuts from burning.

4. Easily remove the walnuts from the pan and place onto a paper towel.
5. Sprinkle with salt.
6. Mix the lettuce and carrots in a bowl. Mix the orange juice and the walnuts before serving.

Rolls Containing Low-Fodmap Spring

Ingredients:

Filling;

- 2 carrot
- Rice paper
- Half a cup of basil
- 2 turnip
- 2 cup of cilantro
- 20 medium-sized shrimps
- Half a cup of mint
- 2 zucchini

Marinate;

- A pinch of white Pepper
- 4 teaspoons of chopped ginger
- 2 tablespoon of garlic infused olive oil
- 2 tablespoon of scallions (green part only)

- 2 teaspoon of fish sauce
- 2 tablespoon of coconut oil
- 4 teaspoons of gluten free soy sauce

- Peanut Sauce;
- 4 tablespoons of wheat free soy sauce
- 4 teaspoons of fish sauce
- 4 tablespoons of freshly squeezed lime juice
- 4 teaspoons of natural cane syrup
- 2 teaspoon of dried chilli flakes
- 4 tablespoons of garlic infused olive oil
- A quarter cup of natural smooth peanut butter (sugar free)

Instruction:

1. To prepare the shrimp by marinating; Easily   put   all   the   marinade ingredients into a ziplock bag, Mix the shrimp and refrigerate for slightly more than thirty-six minutes.

2. Easily put all the ingredients for the peanut sauce into a large mixing bowl and stir with a wooden spoon until well combined.

3. Cut or julienne the turnip, savoy cabbage, and zucchini.

4. Place the coconut oil in a large skillet and sauté the remaining ingredients for 5 to 10 minutes

5. To easy make the spring rolls, place the rice vermicelli in a large bowl of water for 5 to 10 minutes, until it often a bit, then easily remove it along with a portion of the vegetable, cilantro, and hrmr.

6. Next, break the mint leaves and basil by hand and place them in the rolls.

7. Fold in the de, then roll the wraps gently, and voilà! Your own homemade Low-FODMAP spring rolls!

Yummy Warm Chia Pudding

INGREDIENTS

- 4 tablespoons pure maple syrup

- 1 tablespoon cinnamon

- 1 cup chia seeds (black, white, or mix)

- 5 cups unsweetened plain almond milk or oat milk

- 2 teaspoon pure vanilla extract

Quick Caramelized Bananas

- 2 teaspoon coconut oil

- 1/2 teaspoon cinnamon

- 2 banana, cut into slices

- 2 teaspoon pure maple syrup

73

Warmed Berries

- 2 tablespoon pure maple syrup

- 1 cup frozen mixed berries

Directions

1. In a small pot add almond milk, vanilla, maple syrup, cinnamon, and chia seeds and whisk vigourously to combine
2. Set aside and let sit for 35 to 40 minutes to thicken.
3. Once thickened, place pot on the stovetop over medium-high heat and stir continuously to warm throuhout and thicken into a thin pudding consistency.
4. Easily remove from heat and prepare bananas and berries if using for toppings.
5. For the Quick Caramelized Bananas, add the bananas to a sauce pan with the oil, maple syrup, and cinnamon and saute over medium heat until soft and lightly browned about 5-10 minutes.

6. For the Warmed Berries, add the frozen berries and maple syrup to a saucepan over high heat and stir and mash until warmed throughout, soft, and slightly thickened, about 5-10 minutes.
7. DIvide the warm chia pudding between 1-5 bowls or jars and top with the bananas and berries and a sprinkle of nuts and/or seeds.
8. Enjoy while warm!

Chocolate-Mint Bars

Ingredients

- Nonstick cooking spray
- 1/2   cup soy flour 1 cup cornstarch
- 2 teaspoon xanthan gum or guar gum
- 4 heaping tablespoons unsweetened cocoa powder
- 16 tablespoons unsalted butter, cut into cubes, at room temperature
- 1/2   cup superfine sugar
- 1 cup superfine white rice flour

Peppermint Filling

- 8 ounces good-quality dark chocolate, broken into pieces 2 tablespoon plus 2 teaspoon light cream
- 6 scant tablespoons vegetable shortening
- 2 cup confectioners' sugar
- One 8-ounce package reduced-fat cream cheese, at room temperature 6 to 8 teaspoons peppermint extract
- 1 cup plus 2 tablespoons vegetable shortening, melted
- Chocolate Topping

Instructions

1. Set the oven's temperature to 350 °F (200°C). Apply nonstick cooking spray to an 10x5-inch baking sheet and line with parchment paper.
2. Using an electric mixer, combining the butter and sugar in a medium bowl and beat until thick and pale.
3. Sift the cocoa, cornstarch, xanthan gum, soy flour, rice flour, and three times into a separate bowl.
4. With a sizable metal spoon, blend the addition with the butter and sugar that have been creamed.
5. Form a loose ball and just give it a quick knead in the bowl. Into the prepared pan, press the dough–25 to 30 minutes, or up to golden.
6. Place aside and allow to fully cool. Confectioners' sugar, cream cheese, and peppermint essence are

combined to form the peppermint filling.

7. This mixture is then well mixed with a handheld electric mixer.

8. Shortening should be added, then beaten for one to two minutes until smooth.

9. Refrigerate until firm after evenly distributing the mixture over the cookie shell.

10. Dark chocolate, cream, and shortening should be easily put in a small saucepan and heated slowly while being stirred constantly to form the chocolate topping.

11. Spread the chocolate coating over the peppermint filling after just taking the pan out of the fridge.

12. Slice into squares once chilled and ready to serve.

Spread Of Sun-Dried Tomatoes

INGREDIENTS

- 2 tbsp. garlic-infused olive oil
- 6 tbsp. olive oil
- Salt and freshly ground black pepper
- 2 cup sun-dried fresh tomatoes in oil, drained, and roughly chopped 1/2 cup roughly chopped flat-leaf parsley
- 4 heaping tbsp. reduced-fat cream cheese, at room temperature

Directions:

1. Sun-dried tomatoes, preserved oil, parsley, and cream cheese should all be thoroughly combined in a food processor or blender.

2. Once the mixture is nearly smooth, gradually Mix the garlic-infused oil and olive oil.

3. To taste, Mix salt and pepper to the food.

4. Place in a dish or jar, cover, and refrigerate for up to 1-5 days.

Low folate and lactose summer squash soup

Ingredients:

1/2 teaspoon mustard powder

1/2 teaspoon cinnamon

8 cups (2 L) Low FODMAP Vegetable Broth

1/2 cup (2 80 ml) canned whole coconut milk, at room temperature

Kosher salt

Freshly ground black pepper

Cilantro leaves

6 tablespoons Garlic-Infused Oil, made with vegetable oil or olive oil, or purchased equivalent

2 cup (68 g) finely chopped scallions, green parts only

8 cups (600 g) chopped trimmed patty pan squash

8 medium Yukon gold potatoes, peeled and chopped

6 medium carrots, trimmed, peeled and chopped

2 teaspoon cumin powder

2 teaspoon coriander

2 teaspoon turmeric

2 teaspoon paprika, plus extra for garnish

Preparation:

1. Heat a large, heavy-bottomed pot over low-medium heat.
2. Mix the oil and the scallion greens and sauté until softened, but not browned.
3. Mix the squash, potatoes, carrots and all of the spices.
4. Stir together and simple cook for a few minutes or until vegetables just begin to soften.

5. Mix the stock, cover, bring to a boil, then adjust heat and simmer for about 25 to 30   minutes or until all the vegetables are very tender.
6. If you have an immersion blender, you can purée the soup right in the pot.
7. Otherwise, transfer to blender and purée.
8. Return soup to pot, if necessary. Taste and season with salt and pepper.
9. Soup is ready to garnish and serve.
10.   Divide the hot soup into serving bowls, swirl in some coconut milk, garnish with cilantro leaves and a sprinkle of paprika.
11. You can also refrigerate the puréed soup in an airtight container for up to 1-5 days.

Oat And Almond Waffles

- 1 cup rice flour
- 1 cup chopped almonds
- 2 tablespoon baking powder
- 1 teaspoon sea salt
- 1 cups almond or coconut milk
- 2 large egg
- ½ cup olive oil
- 2 cup rolled oats (gluten-free)

1. Heat the waffle maker to a medium-high temperature.
2. Spray the waffle iron liberally with cooking spray or coconut oil.
3. In a small bowl, whisk the almond milk, egg, and olive oil until smooth.
4. In a medium bowl, combine the oats, rice flour, almonds, baking powder, and salt.
5. Stir the egg mixture into the flour mixture until uniform.

6. Pour about 1/3 cup of batter per waffle onto the waffle iron.
7. Close the waffle iron and simple cook for 5 to 10 minutes, until the exterior is golden and crisp and the interior is fully cooked.
8. Repeat until all waffles have been cooked.
9. Serve without delay.

Pizza Breakfast Frittata

Ingredients:

- 1 cup ricotta cheese
- 8 tbsp oil
- ½ tsp nutmeg
- Seasoning to taste
- 20 fresh eggs
- 9oz spinach ripped into smaller pieces
- 2 oz pepperoni
- 2 tsp garlic, minced
- 10 oz mozzarella cheese

Directions:

1. Preheat the oven to 350
2. Blend the fresh eggs, flavors, and oil together
3. Include the cheddar and spinach

4. Mix to some skillet, sprinkle with some additional mozzarella cheddar on top

5. Mix the little pepperoni to easy make it resemble a pizza

6. Easily put in the broiler and prepare for just 60 minutes

7. Present with your most loved greasy dressings.

Potato Pancakes

Ingredients:

.

6 tablespoons oil

¾ cup spring onions (green parts only), chopped

.

1 teaspoon ground black pepper

.2 teaspoon salt

2 1 lbs potatoes, peeled, grated

.4 fresh eggs, beaten

.2 tablespoon all-purpose flour

1. .Squeeze overabundance fluid out of potatoes, a small bunch at a time.

2. In an enormous bowl, place the fresh eggs, flour, onions, salt and pepper.

3. Mix   the   potatoes   and   stir.

4. Pour in 1 tbsp. oil into an enormous non-stick   skillet   and   spot   over medium-high heat.

5. 8 . Scoop the potato blend into your hands and shape into a level flapjack.

6. Place in the skillet, level and fry for 5-10 minutes on each side.

7. Do this with the excess hotcakes and enjoy.

Low Fodmap Tomato Soup With Rsy

INGREDIENTS

- 6 tbsp ginger syrup
- 2 tsp sambal or more to taste (hot chili pepper paste)
- 2 tsp ground ginger
- 4 tbsp corn starch
- 2 00 g rice vermicelli
- 2 liter water
- 4 low FODMAP stock cubes
- 800 g canned peeled fresh tomatoes
- 400 g canned diced tomatoes
- 2 large tin of tomato paste
- 4 tbsp sugar
- 4 tbsp soy sauce
- Optional: one stalk spring onion for garnish

INSTRUCTIONS

1. Bring one liter of water and two stoichiometric cubes to a boil.
2. Mix tomato paste and peeled tomatoes.
3. Bring to a boil again.
4. Combine the sugar, soy sauce, ginger syrup, ginger powder, and sambal in a bowl.
5. Mix to the soup and mix thoroughly.
6. Mix salt to the soup in order to enhance its flavor.
7. If you like uour soup a bit more srisu, uou can Mix some extra sambal.
8. Do this in very small amounts, one teaspoon at a time, or else your mouth will become extremely spicy and painful.
9. Use a hand blender to transform the liquid into a smooth liquid.

10. Combine the sorn tartar sauce and 12 tablespoons of water in a small bowl and stir until smooth.
11. Mix to the our and mix well.
12. Fnallu incorporate the rice vermicelli and bean sprouts into the our.
13. Allow the soup to simmer for an additional 1-5 minutes.

Pina Colada Bites

INGREDIENTS:

- 2 tablespoon of liquid glucose
- 4 teaspoons Coconut extract
- 15 kg pineapple
- 2 1 cups caster sugar
- 2 cup of water

DIRECTIONS:

1. Cut the pineapple slices into smaller bits.
2. Combine the sugars and water into a saucepan, stirring until all the sugars are melted.
3. Bring the liquid to a simmer.
4. Add the pineapple and 4 teaspoons coconut extract.
5. Slowly continue to simmer for 70 to 80 minutes or until the pineapple is opaque.
6. Use a slotted spoon to transfer to a rack placed over a baking tray lined with baking paper.
7. Preheat oven to 250 F. Bake for 2 hours, to dry the pineapple.
8. Allow the pineapple to cool.
9. Store in an airtight container at room temperature or refrigerate if the atmosphere is humid.

Quinoa With Almonds And Feta, Flavored

Ingredients

6 00g quinoa , rinsed

10 0g toasted flaked almonds

2 00g feta cheese, crumbled

handful parsley, roughly chopped

juice 1 lemon

2 tbsp olive oil

2 tsp ground coriander

1 tsp turmeric

Directions

1. Heat the oil in a large pan. Add the spices, then fry for a min or so until fragrant.
2. Add the quinoa, then fry for a further min until you can hear gentle popping sounds.
3. Stir in 600ml boiling water, then gently simmer for 25 to 30 mins until the water has evaporated and the quinoa grains have a white 'halo' around them.
4. Allow to cool slightly, then stir through the
5. other ingredients.
6. Serve warm or cold.

Torte With Chocolate, Cardamom, And Hazelnuts

Ingredients

- 250 g golden caster sugar
- 2 tbsp cocoa powder , plus extra for dusting
- crème fraîche , to serve
- 250 g blanched hazelnuts
- 16 green cardamom pods
- 250 g gluten-free dark chocolate
- 250 g butter
- 12 fresh eggs , separated

Method

1. Toast the hazelnuts in a dry pan until golden, then leave to cool slightly and blitz to a fine consistency in a food processor.
2. Easily remove the cardamom seeds from their pods and grind using a pestle and mortar.
3. Heat oven to 250C fan/gas Grease and line the base of a 40 cm spring-form cake tin.
4. Use a microwave to melt the chocolate with the butter in 60-sec bursts until glossy and smooth.
5. Leave to cool slightly.
6. Using an electric whisk, in a very clean bowl whisk the egg whites until they reach stiff peaks.
7. Then, without cleaning the beaters, whisk the yolks with the sugar in a separate bowl until pale and voluminous.

8. Combine the chocolate with the egg yolk mixture, then incorporate the cocoa powder, a pinch of salt, the cardamom seeds and hazelnuts.

9. Mix a spoonful of egg white to the batter, stirring it through to loosen the mix, then fold in the rest, just taking care to keep in as much air as possible.

10.   Gently pour into the tin and bake for 350 mins.

11.   Leave to cool in the tin, then dust with cocoa powder and serve with crème fraîche.

Millet (Type Cornbread) Bread

- Simple easy make 2 2 portions
- 1 teaspoon sodium carbonate
- 1   tsp salt 250g coconut cream (can)
- 4 tbsp lemon juice
- 4 fresh eggs
- 120g olive oil
- 2 teaspoon of honey (or xylitol)
- 2 teaspoon vanilla, optional
- 260g millet flour 250 g chopped walnuts
- 70 g tapioca flour 70 g cassava flour
- 2 tsp baking powder

1. Line a square 40 cm baking dish with parchment paper.

2. Preheat the oven to 250 degrees Celsius, and mark 5-10 on the gas scale.

3. Place the flour and walnuts in a food processor and pulse until the walnuts are finely ground.

4. Mix the other ingredients and continue beating until a batter forms.

5. Spoon the batter into the prepared pan.

6. 30-40 minutes in the oven will enough.

7. Allow cooling in the pan before slicing it into pieces.

Salad Garden With Carrot-Ginger Dressing

Ingredients

Dressing

1 teaspoon clover honey or pure maple syrup

4 tablespoons mayonnaise

1 teaspoon sea salt

½ cup extra-virgin olive, grapeseed, or avocado oil

4 medium-size carrots peeled and roughly chopped

2 (2-inch) piece fresh ginger, peeled

½ cup sauerkraut or fermented cabbage
(see headnote)

4 tablespoons apple cider vinegar

Salad

2 cup cherry tomatoes, halved, or
4 vine tomatoes, chopped
4 heads romaine lettuce, thinly sliced

2 cup thinly sliced red or green cabbage

2 seedless cucumber, finely diced

Sea salt

2 tablespoons black sesame seeds, for
garnish

Instructions

1. Create the dreng: Combine the potatoes, onions, cabbage, vinegar, honey, mayonnaise, and salt in a food processor or blender until smooth.
2. To nsorrorate, Mix additional oil and whisk.
3. Mix water, 1-5 tablespoons at a time, until the mixture resembles ranch dressing.
4. Set aside or store until ready to just consume.

5. Prepare the salad: Spread the romaine and cabbage on a large platter.

6. The cucumbers and fresh tomatoes should then be arranged on top of the dressing.

7. Lightly season the vegetables with salt and sesame seeds.

8. Serve immediately alongside the remaining dressing.

Penne With Basil-Walnut Pesto
Gluten-Free

2 pound penne pasta (gluten-free) 2 cups basil leaves, neatly packed
 1 cup walnuts, chopped
  1 cup Parmesan cheese, grated
2 /6 cup of garlic oil

1. Over high heat, bring a large saucepan of water to a boil.
2. Simple cook the penne according to package directions until al dente, 5-10 minutes.
3. Meanwhile, in a food processor, finely chop and combine the basil, walnuts, Parmesan, and garlic oil. Don't puree it.
4. Drain the pasta in a colander when it's done.

5. Toss the pesto with the hot spaghetti. Serve right away.

Spinach Ravioli

Ingredients:

2 cup of lactose-free cheese
2 cup of lactose-free yogurt
½ tsp of salt
½ tsp of pepper
4 cups of tapioca flour
2 cup of rice flour
4 cups of water
6 fresh eggs
6 egg whites
12 tbsp of olive oil
4 cups of spinach, chopped

Preparation:

1. In a large bowl, combine tapioca and rice flour, water, fresh eggs, egg whites, olive oil and a pinch of salt.

2. You really want to easy make a smooth dough.

3. Cover and let it stand in a warm place for about 60 minutes.

4. Briefly boil spinach in salted water, drain and cut.

5. Combine with lactose-free cheese, lactose-free yogurt, salt and pepper.

6. Roll the dough thinly, cut out circles using molds and easily put in each hemisphere spoon of stuffing.

7. Just replace the second part of dough and press the edges with a fork so that the stuffing does not fall off.

8. Simple cook ravioli in boiling water to which you have added a little salt and olive oil.

9. It should take about 30 minutes.

10.   Easily remove from the saucepan, drain and serve.

Conclusion

I hope that this book was able to assist you in living a life free of IBS symptoms by eliminating FODMAP from your diet.

The next step is to immediately eliminate all high FODMAP foods and condiments from your home and just replace them with low FODMAP alternatives. You deserve a life free from the misery that is IBS. Begin the low FODMAP diet immediately!

www.ingramcontent.com/pod-product-compliance
Lightning Source LLC
Chambersburg PA
CBHW060527030426
42337CB00015B/2000